ESHU-ELEGBARA

SANTERIA AND THE
ORISHA OF THE CROSSROADS

BY BABA RAUL CANIZARES

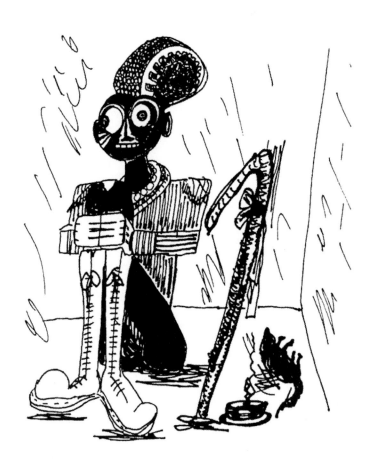

ORIGINAL PUBLICATIONS

ESHU - ELEGGUA

SANTERIA AND THE ORISHA OF THE CROSSROADS

© 2000 by ORIGINAL PUBLICATIONS

ISBN: 0-942272-61-7

Original Publications
P.O. Box 236
Old Bethpage, New York 11804-0236
1-888-OCCULT-1

Printed in the United States of America

1

INTRODUCTION

*"Eshu throws a stone today
and kills a bird yesterday"*

Amid the hustle and bustle of Havana's Rancho Boyeros International Airport, a young woman excitedly waits in line to board the small plane that will take her to fame. Young and beautiful, cabaret singer Roxana Gonzalez had been chosen to lead a troupe of Cuban performers on a triumphal tour of Central and South America. This was the moment she had been waiting for since she was ten years old and had won first prize in a radio show called "Searching for Stars" --this was fifty years before Ed McMahon made a similar show famous on American TV

Roxana giggled with her girlfriends, the four platinum-blonde beauties that made up the musical group *"Las Platinadas de Oscar Moreno."* All of a sudden, a serious-looking black youth wearing an impeccably laundered and ironed red shirt and black pants approached Roxana and, staring straight into her face, told her, "Senora, don't go." Startled, the young artist turned to her friends: "Did you hear what that kid say?" Staring at her with a puzzled look on her face, one of her friends asked her, "What kid? I didn't see anybody!" Roxana looked around, but the child had vanished. Panicking, Roxana left the line. "I'm not going on that plane, and you should do the same," she told her friends. The impressario overheard what Roxana said and ordered her to get on the plane, or she would miss her performance in Panama. "I'll take a later flight, but I'm not getting on that plane." Now red with rage the impressario, a very influential man, told Roxana that unless she got on that plane he'd make sure she never worked again. Sad but determined, Roxana went back home. The next morning she was awakened by her mother with the horrifying news that the plane had gone down and there had been no survivors. Cuba went into mourning for some of the most talented young performers it had, all dead in a plane crash. This was 1953. Two years before I was born. Roxana Gonzalez was my mother, who went on to raise a family, passing away in 1994. My mother was convinced that the child that saved her life was none other than Eshu, the orisha of the crossroads. Had she not heeded his advice, I wouldn't be here today, writing these lines.

Eshu, called "Eleggua" in Santeria, is one of the deities of the Yoruba pantheon (The Yoruba people formed a nation which today is part of the modern republic of Nigeria). These deities share striking similarities with gods and goddesses of other cultures. This has led some students of Yoruba religion to refer to them as Jungian[1] archetypes. A Jungian archetype is a prototypic phenomenon that simultaneously forms part of the so-called collective unconscious and is accessible to each individual's unconscious. Since these archetypes are believed to reflect human thoughts regardless of place, time, or culture, proponents of equating the orisha with these archetypes argue that in this manner, people outside the orisha-worshipping community who are familiar with Jung's work may gain an understanding of the orisha.[2]

Yoruba theology teaches that there are 401 powers of the right ("angels") called orisha whose role is to act as protectors and facilitators of humankind; there are also 201 powers of the left called ajogun ("demons") whose role is to present humans with challenges and obstacles. Eshu's place is unique because he is both an orisha and the leader of the ajogun! He is the "one" in four-hundred-and-one and the one in two-hundred-and-one. As head ajogun, Eshu commands the eight warlords of the left, agents of mischief Iku (death), Arun (sickness), Egba (paralysis), Epe (curse), Ewon (imprisonment), Oran (big trouble), Ofo (big loss), and Ese (all other problems). For this reason, Eshu is as feared as he is loved. Eshu is offered sacrifice before any other orisha in every ceremony[3], he is unique in that everywhere where the orisha are worshipped, Eshu is honored. manifestations are countless, his attributes many. In Cuba he is generally called Eleggua. Although it is commonly believed that Eleggua is a mispronunciation of Elegbara, one of Eshu's many manifestations in Africa, the tradition in my lineage is that Eleggua is the Hispanicized form of Elewa, a praise name for Eshu meaning "handsome one." This makes sense since one finds numerous instances of Lukumi writers in Cuba substituting "g" for "w."[4] Eshu is considered the god of fate and as such can be said to be the most important orisha. His ability to facilitate one's aspirations, as well as his being able to block them, makes him indispensable: Simply stated, without Eshu nothing can be accomplished!

2

"PATAKI"
SACRED STORIES
ABOUT ESHU

A "Pataki" is a holy tale about the Orisha. These sacred stories, passed down from generation to generation, make up an orally transmitted corpus of hagiographies possessing great beauty and timeless lessons. When a practitioner casts the sixteen-cowry oracle called "merindilogun," the number of shells that fall with their natural opening facing up determines which of these pataki⁵ are to be recited. Within these sacred stories, answers to problems presented to the orisha for solutions are to be found. Because of Eshu's unequaled importance, there are more pataki about him than about any other orisha. What follows are but a few of the thousands of stories about the divine trickster

Birth stories: In his most basic form, Eshu is eternal, he is thought not to have had a beginning and will not have an end, but many of his avatars have experienced birth and death. The following pataki is often told in Cuba.⁶

It is said that many, many years ago there lived in Africa a righteous monarch named Okubere who had a wife named Ananaki. After years of marriage, the couple began to worry because Ananaki had not been able to conceive. Unlike other kings of the region, Okubere refused to have other wives, being very much in love with Ananaki. Ananaki pleaded with the king to divorce her so he could marry a woman who could give him an heir, or to take a secondary wife as was his right as a king. Okubere, however, refused to accept either of those solutions, preferring to stay put with his beloved Ananaki. One moonless night, thinking she was doing Okubere a favor, Ananaki ran away from the royal compound, leaving her husband free to marry someone else. Ananaki walked and walked until fatigue overcame her and she fell down on the ground, completely exhausted. A huge coconut fell from a nearby palm. It was an enormous fruit, bright green and shiny. Ananaki stood up and walked towards the palm, picking up the coconut and cracking it with a stone in order to drink its delicious juice. Ananaki then laid down by the palm tree and fell asleep. "Ananaki! Ananaki!" The woman awoke, hearing a strong voice calling her name. "It is I, Ananaki, the Coconut Palm Tree! You have drunk of my blood, which has made your womb fertile, many children will be nurtured in that womb, but if you do not wish to lose the first one, you must dedicate him to me three days after he is born. He will be blessed with great beauty and intelligence, and God Almighty will make him Lord of the Road." Too shocked to say a word, Ananaki stood up and hurried back to her husband.

Ananaki found Okubere crying his eyes out for her, desolate after looking all over for his beloved Ananaki without luck. Ananaki told her husband what had transpired and he rejoiced in the knowledge that he and his wife would be able to conceive. "Blessed be the Coconut Palm Tree!"--Shouted the king. Nine months to the day of Ananaki's return, a beautiful boy was born to the pair. So great was their joy that both forgot all about the Coconut Palm Tree. They named their boy Eleggua, which in their tongue means "handsome one." Prince Eleggua was the apple of everyone's eyes, and he grew strong, handsome, and somewhat spoiled. Going hunting one day with his entourage, young Eleggua felt a strange chill go up his spine when he got to the middle of a certain crossroads. He stopped dead in his tracks with a strained, anguished expression on his face, worrying his hunting companions who had never seen the rambunctious youngster act so strangely. After a couple of minutes that seemed like hours to his worried followers, Eleggua bent down to pick up something from the ground. It was a strange, luminous coconut. The prince seemed to be fascinated by it, carefully carrying it back home.

Showing his parents the fruit, they laughed and said they saw nothing unusual about it. Eleggua then rolled the coconut on the floor, the thing ending up in a corner by the front door of his chamber. One day, not long after the incident with the coconut, the king offered a great feast to celebrate Eleggua's birthday when a powerful, blinding light began to issued from Eleggua's room. Investigating the phenomenon, the king's bodyguard discovered that the source of the light was the coconut by the prince's doorway. Many of the king's guests left the party, utterly terrified. The king ordered that the coconut should be offered obeisances, as it was obviously a divine emanation. Three days later, however, an inconceivable tragedy befell the village when their beloved prince Eleggua fell ill and died suddenly. Everyone felt the loss of the handsome youth. While the prince's body lay in state, the coconut kept his chamber, now transformed into a funeral parlor, fully illuminated. After the Prince's burial, however, everyone forgot about the coconut, which lay forgotten behind the dead prince's door.

After Eleggua's death, the village fell into a downward spiral where nothing prospered; cows refused to give milk, chickens refused to eat, and plants refused to grow. King Okubere called all the great diviners of his realm and beyond to find the cause of his village's misfortune. The wise men, through divination, found out that the reason for the village's adversity, and also the reason for the young prince's death, lay in the royal couple's forgotten promise to the Coconut Palm Tree. "You must offer obeisance to the magic coconut, or we will all starve!" The seers told the king. Unfortunately, when they went to look for the fruit, they found that it had rotted away and was no good. They then took what was left of the coconut and, finding a suitable stone (one as large and round as the coconut), they smeared the fleshy pulp, now soft and gooey from rot, on the surface of the stone. They then sacrificed a beautiful white rooster, brought in from another village, on top of the stone, which they further dressed with honey and palm oil. By divination they found out that the spirit of the magic coconut now occupied the stone. Okubere and Ananaki proceeded to lovingly install the stone behind the door of Eleggua's chamber. The stone then began to glow. Through teary eyes the grief-stricken parents saw an ethereal, translucent face begin to appear over the stone. It was the face of their ill-fated son, Eleggua. They then understood that they had not lost their son, who had become an orisha and would now be protecting them from his divine realm. Eventually, the wise elders taught Okubere and Ananaki how to communicate with Eleggua by using an oracle consisting of four pieces of coconut. Since that day everyone in the community enjoyed great prosperity. Eventually, each household in the village had its own Eleggua stone prepared so that Eleggua's cult became widespread, eventually being adopted by other villages until every corner of the world had heard the name Eleggua, the magical prince who became a god.

Commentary: This pataki is considered very important because it encapsulates one of the most sacred tenets of Santeria: That the dead precede the orisha. Here we clearly see how Eleggua was first human before dying and subsequently becoming an orisha. Although Eleggua is the first orisha to be propitiated, the ancestors, the egungun, are honored even before Eleggua.

Why Eleggua eats first: There are many pataki that relate why Eleggua is the first orisha to be propitiated, the following is the most commonly related in Cuba.

Once upon a time, long before there was a separation between humans and Orisha, Obatala lived in a splendid palace with his wife Yemmun and their children, the eldest of them being the strong and righteous Ogun. Baba, as Obatala is called by all creation, took pleasure in his serious, diligent offspring. In those days Baba was very much a hands-on ruler, his meticulous attention to all corners of his vast empire taking him away from home when he felt his subjects in those places needed him. It was during one of these sojourns of Obatala that Ogun began to feel a shameful attraction for his own mother. Obatala had an enchanted rooster named Ósun[7] that served as his eyes and ears while he was away. Determined to consummate his shameful desire towards Yemmu, Ogun machinated a diabolical plan to possess her. He first overfed the rooster, giving him his own brother Eleggua's portion of food. Eleggua in this incarnation was a little boy. The bloated Ósun proceeded to fall into a morbid slumber. Ogun then put his little brother out, locking the door so he couldn't re-enter the house. With the coast clear, Ogun consummated the incest.[8]

Ogun and Yemmu's opprobrious act continued each time Baba was away. On one occasion as the family sat for dinner, Obatala noticed how gaunt and rueful his little Eleggua looked. Calling him to the side, Obatala asked the youngster, "Tell me, son, what is wrong? Why are you so thin? Why are your eyes cloudy?" Measuring his words, sorry for the pain he was to cause his beloved Baba, but aware that the shame had to end, Eleggua told Obatala: "Father, each time you go away Ogun feeds my portion of food to Ósun, who then goes to sleep. Ogun then locks me out of the house and stays inside alone with Mother." Horrified at the thought that was darkening his mind, Obatala decided not to say anything at that time, but to conduct a test. He announced that he would be gone for several days and appeared to ride away on his horse, as he had done many times before. Surreptitiously, however, Obatala turned right back and hid where he could see the front of his compound. He witnessed as Ogun locked Eleggua out and overfed Ósun. Obatala then entered his home seeing the most heinous act a husband and father can witness. Horrified at the presence of his father, Ogun for the first time felt the full weight of his sin. Covering his face in shame, Ogun cried "Do not curse me father, for I curse myself, from this day on I shall labor day and night, never will my body experience the comfort of rest. The secret of making iron tools and weapons, which I have so zealously guarded, will I give to humanity, so not longer the Lord of the Forge will I be, and worst of all, I shall never see my beloved family again, I'll live like an animal in the deepest jungle." "And so it shall be!" declared the Father. Turning to Eleggua, Baba said, "From this day forth you will be served before anyone else, and you will be worshipped before any god! Unless you eat first, no one else will eat." Turning to the rooster, Baba said: "And you, Ósun, because you have betrayed me for food, will only eat the scraps Eleggua throws your way, and you will live only to serve him." And so it was that sin entered the world, due to a son's forbidden love for his mother.

Commentary: This pataki clearly establishes Eleggua's primacy over all orisha. It also serves to illustrate how sin entered the world. As in the Garden of Eden myth, a disobedient son and sexual misconduct are the elements that disrupted an idyllic existence, but out of this tragedy, something precious was obtained for humankind: the knowledge of how to work iron into useful objects of war and industry!

Oshun, Oya, and Yemaya become "Psychic Readers": Another Pataki that establishes Eleggua's primacy concerns a time when Oshun, Oya, and Yemaya decided to set up a joint practice as "psychic readers"--actually, cowry shell casters. The sisters hired Eleggua to serve as their publicist and manager. Pooling their resources, the group bought a nice little cottage near the ocean. "You get the clients in here, and we'll split our take four ways!" Said Yemaya to Eleggua Laroye, who in this avatar has "the gift of the gab." No sooner did Eleggua Laroye begin to pass the word around that the three greatest cowry shell readers in the world had set up shop on the beach that hundreds of clients began to appear at the sisters' door, anxious to have their fortunes told. At the end of each day Eleggua would come by the cottage to collect his bounty. After about three months, Oya began to protest having to give so much money to Eleggua. "After all, we do all the work!," the queen of the dead said.[9] The sisters agreed that, with so many clients, they didn't need Eleggua anymore. From then on, each evening Eleggua would pass by the sisters' cottage only to be told "Nothing today, son, it's been a very slow day, but try tomorrow and we'll see." After a week of this, Eleggua stood close to the cottage, on the only road which led to the sisters. Each time a client would approach, Eleggua would send him or her away saying "the sisters don't live in the cottage anymore, but leave me your address and I'll let you know their new whereabouts as soon as I know it myself."

After a few days Oshun, Oya, and Yemaya began to panic as they saw day in and day out without any business being transacted. Yemaya demanded to know why Eleggua wasn't keeping his end of the deal. "Have you?," asked Eleggua impassively. Lowering her gaze, Yemaya realized that she and her sisters had not acted fairly with Eleggua. "From now on your cut will be the first we separate from the day's intake."--Yemaya said--" in fact, from now on I'll make sure your plate of food is the first served, and your clothes are the first washed." After Yemaya and Eleggua made the pact that assured Eleggua his primacy, everything went back to normal. Since that time it has become customary to propitiate Eleggua first.

Commentary: This pataki is unusual in that it treats cowry shell reading very much as a business. The Yoruba did not view religion as separate from their everyday lives, for this reason they found nothing wrong with a practitioner who spends his or her time counseling others being remunerated for it. The obvious moral of this tale, however, is the need to keep one's promises and contracts, and the righteousness of acting fairly.

Eshu red and black: There were two friends who grew up together in a small, West African village. They did everything together since they were very young. Both attended the same classes, served the army at the same time, and bought adjoining farms when they were ready to settle down. They even married on the same day. The two friends were so close they never even had an argument. Once they went to see a babalawo to check on the state of their affairs, as was the custom in their village. The babalawo told the friends that unless they made a sacrifice to Eshu, they would have a great fight between them. The friends disrespected the babalawo by laughing in his face: "We, have a fight? Not likely!" the two men said. Needless to say, they refused to make sacrifice to Eshu. Sometime later the two buddies were tilling the soil on each side of the narrow trail that separated their respective properties, when a man passed by, offering them a quick greeting as he walked by at a rather fast pace. "I wonder who that was," one of the friends said to the other. "I don't know, but I can't imagine how he can stand the heat dressed in black like that" The other friend responded. "What do you mean black, dear friend? He was all in red, from head to feet!" "Red?"--Asked the other one--"You clown! You know very well he was dressed in black, and he seemed to be crying" The friend who said he saw the man dressed in red now turned sullen. "Are you calling me a liar, beloved one? He wore red and was laughing!" "Are YOU calling me a liar, highly valued comrade?" The friends' first argument ever escalated into a horrible brawl, where neighbors had to come and separate them. Such anger erupted between them that they flipped a coin to decide who would leave town.

Twenty years passed by when each of the former friends received a message from the Chief of the Temple of Eshu at the royal palace to offer sacrifice there. Honored by such a request, since both were men of modest means, each bought the finest goat he could afford to offer to the trickster god. At the appointed time, the friend who had seen the mysterious man in black twenty years before was instructed to enter the temple through the western door. The other friend was told to enter through the eastern door. In the dimly lit chamber the Chief Priest knelt in front of what seemed to be a magnificent life-size figure of the Lord of the Crossroads. "Come up to the front, both of you," the Priest commanded. Fascinated by the life-size statue, the friends who had not seen each other in twenty years almost bumped into each other as both stared right into the statue, which they now could see was dressed in red and black.

At that moment, what they had thought was a statue stood up, seemingly coming to life. "Welcome, boys, it has been a long time, hasn't it?" Realizing that they were in the presence of Lord Eleggua himself, both men fell on their face in full prostration. "You weren't so worshipful when I passed by your properties twenty years ago, now were you?." Horrified, both friends now saw each other and Eleggua half dressed in red and half in black, right down the middle of his body. The friends realized what a huge mistake they had made and fell down each other's arms sobbing uncontrollably. "Forgive me, beloved friend!" "How could I have been so thoughtless!" The priest offered Eleggua the friends' belated sacrifice and the two friends walked arm in arm with twenty years of stories to share with each other.

Commentary: The moral of this pataki is: Do not be fooled by appearances alone, for appearances may be deceiving. The greater implication is that we should be broad-minded and must strive to see beyond the confines of our own perspective; in doing so, we will be more fully approaching a more complete reality, in the process of which we will be operating closer to the truth of any given situation. As usual with any pataki involving Eleggua, this one reminds us of the importance of making sure we give Eshu what is his without delay.

How Eleggua healed God Almighty: Back in the days when Olodumare was preparing his departure from Earth, leaving his children the Orisha to take over the role of active gods of this planet, something unthinkable occurred, Father Olodumare, God Almighty himself fell ill! This confused all of the Orisha, because they were under the impression that the Great One was incapable of experiencing sickness. Laying in his luxuriant silk blankets, the usually vital Patriarch seemed to be ebbing away. One by one, all the Orisha tried to heal God using everything they knew, one by one they failed. Obatala and Olokun, God's two most powerful children, began preparations to face the unthinkable: The death of God. Ifa, destiny personified, divined that there was one orisha they had all forgotten to consult: Eshu Beleke, a tiny, onerous, childlike Orisha who enjoyed living where refuse was gathered or deep in the jungle. Because of his strange appearance and nasty disposition, Eshu Beleke had been ostracized by his fellow Orisha, which suited him fine since he preferred to be alone anyway.

Oshosi Ode Mata, the Hunt personified, was sent to track Eshu Beleke down. Sure enough, the tiny terror was found in a squalid garbage dump near a small village. "Greetings, honorable brother," Oshosi said. Eating a piece of decaying rat, Eshu didn't even bother to look up, simply telling Oshosi to go f--k himself. "I do not mean to disturb your meditation, Eshu, but our Father has fallen ill and we have all tried everything we know to heal him without success, you are our last hope." "Of course you can't heal him, the only cure for what ails Olodumare is to be found here, in the squalor of a garbage dump, and of course none of you highbrow mother f-----s with your noses all up in your asses would be caught dead near garbage, but all right, I'll heal him. Its not his fault all of you are a pack of losers." The small figure then began to rapidly gather some herbs from the malodorous waste. Eshu then triturated the herbs to a fine powder, mixing the powder with some cloudy liquid he had in a container. Eshu then proceeded to give the mixture to Olodumare, who almost instantly after drinking it returned to full health.

So overjoyed was God with Eshu that he decreed that from then on all other orisha would have to defer to him, allowing him to be propitiated first at all ceremonies, and asking for his blessing before embarking on any endeavor. Eshu became God's own messenger and the Lord of the Crossroads. He also became the Orisha who, through his Lordship over the Ajogun, agents of mischief, would present humanity with its greatest challenges. All of these boons were more than deserved by the Orisha who saved God Almighty's life!

Commentary: Here we have still another "Why Eleggua eats first" story, yet this one is pregnant with fascinating tidbits of thought provoking wisdom. It posits, for example, that no being is truly immortal, not even God. It warns not to overlook anything, for the most precious substances may be found in the most unlikely places. It also teaches us not to underestimate people nor take them for granted, for no one knows when the talents of the most unlikely people may be of use. At another level, the pataki also teaches us to take advantage of situations and grab the chance to demonstrate our knowledge when the opportunity presents itself.

How Eshu became a babalawo: Olokun, the immensely rich owner of the ocean depths, had a son named Omokun who had the habit of asking Eleggua to bow down before him "because I am a great prince," the young man would say. As it happened, Omokun's dream was to learn the secrets of Ifa divination, but Orunla, the great teacher of Ifa, would not bother with the arrogant youth. Getting tired of the young man's impertinence, the trickster Orisha devised a plan to get back at him. Knowing of Omokun's admiration for Ifa diviners, Eleggua decided to become one.

Arriving at Orunla's house, Eleggua offered him the traditional greeting: "Aboru bora boshishe, Father." "What can I do for you, Eleggua?" The old man asked. "For starters, you can initiate me into the mysteries of Ifa." Startled at first, Orunla smiled, thinking the eternally-youthful Eleggua, known for never keeping much money, was joking. "You know how expensive it is to make Ifa, son, but I'll give you a nice beaded bracelet for free!" "I want you to initiate me as a babalawo, and I want you to do it now!" Apetebi, Orunla's wife., had overheard everything and now interrupted the conversation-something she almost never did unless she perceived her kindhearted husband was being taken advantage of. "You must be crazy, young man, you must have been smoking that ewe-bars herb you're so fond of! It costs one hundred sixteen thousand cowry shells to make Ifa. Work, save your money, and come back in a few years and Father will initiate you." Without saying another word Eleggua climbed to the top of the roof of Orunla's house, throwing himself head first into the hard ground outside. Eleggua lay there unconscious, bleeding profusely. "Oh my God! Oh my God! Do something, Orunla," a flustered Apetabi said. Very worried. Orunla said: "I must give him Ifa initiation right away to save his life!" After initiation ceremonies were performed, Eleggua healed. He stayed with Orunla several months; because of his superior intelligence, Eleggua became a babalawo much faster than a normal person would.

Eleggua placed himself on a road he knew Omokun usually took. When the pretentious young man passed by, he immediately asked Eleggua to bow down. "Perhaps it is you who should bow down before me, for I am a babalawo." Letting out a loud laugh, Omokun said "And where did you get the money to pay for the initiation?" "That doesn't concern you, but I'll prove to you that I am a babalawo. If I weren't a diviner, would I know just by casting this chain that behind your house there is a large tree that you like to admire when you have your morning meal alone, in your room?" Unimpressed, Omokun said "Try another one! Any one of my servants could have given you that bit of information." "All right, how about this one. This morning, upon waking up with an erection, you masturbated thinking of your fifteen-year-old sister, feeling very guilty afterwards. Opening his eyes like saucers, Omokun fell on his knees begging Eleggua to initiate him into the mysteries of Ifa. "All right, then. It'll cost you four-hundred-thousand-sixty-four cowry shells. Since Omokun's father owned the bottom of the ocean, it was no problem for him to come up with the huge sum. Eleggua initiated Omokun and was forever to be venerated by him as his initiating priest. Eleggua then went to see Orunla, giving him half his earning, two-hundred thousand-thirty-two cowry shells, exactly twice the sum Orunla wanted to charge him for making Ifa!

Commentary: This pataki shows the trickster orisha at his best, exhibiting his mischievous justice at work. He had fun forcing the serious Orunla to give him initiation for free only to later on pay him twice the amount Orunla had wanted in the first place. He makes the proud Omokun be forever junior to him by becoming his initiating priest, but makes Omokun's dream of becoming a diviner possible by conferring the Ifa priesthood on him. Eleggua's actions in this story demonstrate why he is Santeria's adorable rascal. Since Eleggua's manifestations are literally countless, it would take several thousand books to begin to compile all of them. In this slim volume we've but scratched the surface of the fascinating character of the Lord of Choices.

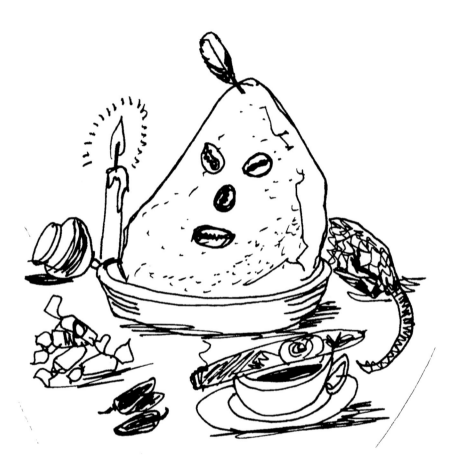

Rock Eleggua with offerings

3

"ONA ESHU"
PATHS OF ELEGGUA

Cuban babalawo Adrian de Souza-Hernandez has noted in his superlative tome on Eshu, "Echu-Eleggua: Equilibrio Dinamico de la Existencia (Habana/Ediciones union, 1998, p.37), "Each artifact or being has its own Eshu." Although most traditions in Cuban Santeria teach that Eshu/Eleggua has twenty-one paths (manifestations, avatars), this figure must be taken as symbolic. Each odu (chapter) in the Ifa corpus has its own Eshu; this alone brings the total to two hundred-fifty-six. Add to that number the many manifestations of the trickster orisha which have come up in the different Diasporic Orisha worshipping populations in the New World and you end up with innumerable personifications of Eshu.

Roads of Eshu in Cuban Santeria: In her excellent work on Orisha worship in Cuba, *Los Orishas en Cuba,* ethnographer Natalia Bolivar Arostegui, who studied under preeminent recorder of Afro-Cuban life Lydia Cabrera, mentions the following paths known in Cuba:

Eleggua Abaile: A messenger avatar, the one who helps with cleansing and decides where to dispose of sacrificial remains.

Eshu Ashi Kuelu: An old man of small stature who lives underground in tunnels and grottoes. He likes gold and is one of the few manifestations that accepts pigeon sacrifices. According to Bolivar, he is the Eshu of the Ifa Odu Owonrin.

Eleggua Afra: The path that accompanies Babalu Aiye, of Dahomeyan "Arara"[10] origin. His colors are black and white, rather than black and red. Does not accept offerings of palm wine or rum; he likes white wine. This Eleggua is fond of whistling around corners. Another path having identical attributes as Afra is called Eshu Makenu.

Eshu Afrodi and Eshu Agroi: Both are Arara Eshus, each is said to have twenty-four paths. They are prepared with twenty-four cowry shells. They look like small pyramids topped by crowns. Priests of Fa (Ifa in Benin) prepare these Eshus; women are not allowed to work with them.

Eleggua Agbanukue Agbanukue: Also from the land of the Arara. A very helpful Eshu. He punishes his enemies by striking them blind.

Eshu Abalonke: Presents himself as a strong adult male, burns his enemies to a crisp, he is said to be an Eshu who walks with Death. This Eshu is born in the Ifa odu Obara Meji.

Eshu Agberu: A female Eshu, sometimes said to be manifested in the terra cotta receptacle where a male Eshu is placed, thus forming a similar representation as the Hindu Yoni-Lingam, the union of male and female in the act of coitus.

Eshu Agbo Bara: A trickster who enjoys gossip.

Eshu Agganika: Dangerous because he is extremely vengeful and unforgiving. He is represented as a soldier on horseback, with a drawn saber.

Eleggua Aggo Meyo: From Oyo. A very efficient solver of major problems.

Eshu Agongo Olo Ona: Lord of the Roads.

Eleggua Agongo Ogo: This is the Eleggua that is represented by a heavy staff.

Eleggua Akeru: A messenger Eleggua.

Eleggua Akesan: Also from Oyo.

Eshu Akileyo: An Eleggua from Oyo characterized as a very badly behaved, hyperactive, little boy.

Eshu Akokor Obiya Akokoriye: From the land of the Mina. He enjoys playing with tops and smoking cigarettes, he is always searching for fun. He also likes to play with a ball.

Eshu Ala Le Ilu: An urban Eshu, old and respected.

Eshu Ala Akomako (Eshu Mako): The Eshu that likes to hide things. He loves to receive stolen offerings; he punishes with fire.

Eshu Ala Ayiki, Bara Alayiki Agaga: This Oyo Eshu eats a lot. Represented by a rambunctious child who loves to party. An incurable alcoholic, Ala Ayiki is said to rule over the Unforeseen. This Eshu is born in the Ifa Odu Ogunda-bosun.

Eleggua Ala La Banshe: Ruler of "That-Which-Will-Come-To-Pass." God gave him the power to makes things go wrong and to right them again, he is, therefore, an indispensable Orisha.

Eshu Alabwana: One of the most important avatars of Eshu, syncretized in Cuba with the Lonely Soul of Purgatory, a medieval Catholic personification of all the suffering souls of that temporary hell. Alabwana is the leader of the egun (dead ancestors). This Eshu is a hermit who lives in the most desolate parts of the wilderness. He is fond of sleeping at the crossroads. Alabwana rules over Win (fairies) and Oyiyi Oku (forest ghosts). It was Alabwana who helped Babalu Aiye when he fell out of favor with Olodumare.

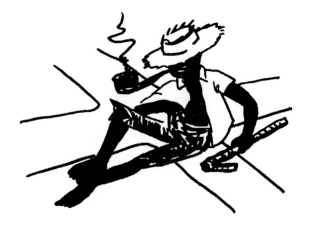

Eshu Alaketu: A former king of Ketu. His colors are black and white.

Eshu Laroye: The most widely worshipped Eshu in Santeria. As Lord of Speech and Communications he is indispensable to effect all interactions between humans and Orisha. A great friend of Oshun, he is also a warrior and is often accompanied by Ogun and Ochosi. He likes offerings of sweets, roosters, and mice.

Eshu Laroye Kio: This is the Eshu that has only one foot.

Eshu Alaru: The Divine Doorman, also a messenger Eshu.

Eshu Alimu: Another Arara Eshu that walks with Babalu.

Eshu Alosi: The closest thing to a devil in Yoruba religion. This Eshu is said to enjoy inflicting pain and suffering, though he only punishes those God has singled out as deserving it. In this way, he is the "left hand of God." The name "Alosi" actually means "Lord of the Left."

Eshu Anaki, Ananaki: Mother of Elegbara, said to have three manifestations, including Eshu Alayi Ibere Yeye, primordial mother of all of the Eshus; As the wife of Eshu Okuboro she is a warrior; she is said to be Wisdom *personified* and is represented by a coconut. As Ayan Bi Lade she is made with one-hundred-one cowry shells, and as Eshu Yangi "she" becomes a "he" and is represented by a laterite stone.

Eshu Ara Idi: An Arara Eshu related to the worship of Oshun and the Ibeji (divine twins).

Eshu Arai Lele: A terrifying Eshu who shape-shifts into a large, fierce dog.

Eshu Arayeyi: Orunla's secretary, protector of Oshun. He is kept near a home's front door.

Eshu Arere Obi Oke: Syncretized in Cuba with the child Jesus held by St. Anthony. A very beneficent Eshu, Olodumare sent him to serve humankind.

Eshu Aridiyi: Loves to scare people.

Eshu Aroni: A healer and magician, he has a very short fuse and is easily irritable. He helps keep Ogun's forge lit. He is a one-armed, one-legged dwarf with a doglike face. This Eshu teaches High Magic, to those brave enough not to be intimidated by him.

Eshu Ayeru: An important defender of Ifa. A babalawo's most trusted guardian.

Eshu Awere: This Eshu lives in the mountains, with Obatala.

Eshu Awo Bara: Another Eshu closely aligned with the practice of Ifa

Eshu Bara Inye: Protects his devotees with fierce passion. This is Shango's Eshu; he appears in the Ifa Odu Obara Meji.

Eshu Barakenyo: The tiniest of Eshus, he is nevertheless very mischievous

Eshu Bara Asuwayo: The Eshu that guards the gates to the holy city of Ile-Ife.

Eshu Bara Layiku: An Eshu from Oyo who helps Babalu with the moving of corpses from one place to another, He also serves as Orunla's doorman. This Eshu can be deadly if not propitiated correctly.

Eshu Baralanugbe: A terrifying avatar who punishes with fire. He is Arara and walks alone. A friend of the Dawn and the Stars.

Eshu Barakinkenyo: A ruthless Child, also called "Obarakikefto."

Eshu Ba Ti Eye, Batiye, Batieye, Batiele: This Eshu is known for his tenacity.

Eshu Beddun Bela: A two-faced Eshu, one being white, the other black.

Eshu Beleke: An Eshu from Ulkumi, he is a naughty child, but he also knows a lot of remedies using herbs. Likes to gossip and to cause misunderstandings. Not a good Eshu for children, for he gets jealous of them.

Eshu Bi Biribi: This Eshu walks with the Ibeji, twin sons of Shango.

Eleggua Biawoona: Fashioned out of stone.

Eshu Bibakikenyo: An Eshu who walks with Oshosi

Eshu Chikua bu: Another Eshu from Oyo, said to be very temperamental.

Eshu Shinki: Lord of Speed

Eshu Shiguidi or Shugudu: His image looks like an inverted cone made of terra cotta, covered with cowry shells. This Eshu is said to cause nightmares. Very rich people and astute businessmen trust Eshu Shiguidi. Shigidi is made by opening a hole in the ground and building him from red clay and offering him blood sacrifices that must be presented in a plate in front of him.

Eshu Daguese: Made out of a large conch.

Eshu Egbayila: A savior Eshu, the Eshu of the Ifa Odu Owanran-Iwori. He is made with gold, silver, platinum and as many different metals as one can find. It also takes palm oil and snake oil, a needle, four straight pins, sand, water from a river, cemetery dirt, dirt from a park, mpembe chalk, toasted corn, red mercury, quicksilver, spurs from a rooster, a piece of goat bone, and sticks from several different trees.

Eshu Elu: Useful as a defensive Eshu, said to be utterly ruthless.

Eshu Elufe: A very fine old gentleman.

Eshu Egbere: Another child Eshu, this one is said to personify the tornado, he walks with Oya.

Eshu Ekileyo: Protector of those seeking wisdom.

Eshu Ere: A two-faced Eshu sculpted out of wood.

Eshu Eshenike: Walks with Osain, is fond of smoking a large pipe filled with herbs.

Eshu Esi Ilenyi: Lives in the front of homes, defender of families.

Eshu Ewe: The Eshu who lives in the forest.

Eshu Guiriyelu: Unlike most other Eshus, this one likes pigeons. saves lives if offered 101 of the feathered creatures as a sacrifice.

Eshu Ina: Fire personified.

Eshu Iyelu: Protects drummers.

Eshu Kakara: Is made inside a conch.

Eshu Kakugbo: Also made with a conch.

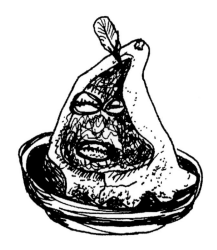

Shell (conch) Eleggua

Eshu Olo Kako Alagada: Likes to play tricks.

Eshu Ka Oloya: An Eshu that lives in the market.

Eshu Kekeno: An Arara Eshu that walks with Babalu.

Eshu Keti: Same as above.

Eshu Kinkeye: Another child manifestation.

Eshu Kolofo: An evil Eshu.

Eshu La Boni: An Eshu who walks with Oshun.

Eshu La To Opa: A wooden Eshu.

Eshu Lawona: An Eshu that seems to be everywhere, allotting punishment to those who deserve it.

Eshu Luyi: An Eshu fashioned inside a conch.

Eshu Marimaye: Doorman of the cemetery.

Eshu Merin Ba Aye: Owner of the crossroads.

Eshu Oba Kere: Eshu as a young king.

Eshu Obasin: Walks with Oduduwa.

Eshu Odemassa: A capricious and bad-tempered Eshu.

Eshu Ode Mata: An Eshu of the forest, companion of Oshosi.

Eshu Odubele: A two-faced Eshu, red on one side, black on the other.

Eshu Oguanni Lele Alaroye: An Eshu that walks with Ogun.

Eshu Owani Legbe: Said to contain the twenty-one boons of the major, paths of Eshu.

Eshu Elegbara: Owner of Strength, believed by many scholars to be the source of the Lukumi word "Eleggua."

Eshu Ogguiri: An Arara Eshu, adopted son of Ajaguna.

Eshu Okada: The Eshu of the garbage, one of his praise names is "Eshu whose penis is like a machete."

Eshu Okuboro: A king, said to be the elder of Elegbara.

Eshu Okokoye Biye: An adult manifestation said to be an orphan from Oyo, raised in the neighboring land of the Mina.

Eshu Olanki (Olonki); Eshu AkokorObiya; Eshu Osika: Three Mina Eshus that always walk together.

Eshu Oni Bode: This Eshu is enshrined as guardian of the metaphysical or actual entrances to certain villages.

Eshu Onini Buruku: A harbinger of death.

Eshu Osa Ika: Eshu of the odu of the same name.

Eshu Sokere: The Eshu of the divining mat.

Eshu Osa Lo Fabeyo: This is an Eshu born in the odu "Osa." He eats pigeons.

The following are paths about which all that is known (to Bolivar) is their name:

Eleggua Agatigaga	Eshu Eleggua Bankeo	Eshu Odara
Eleggua Agbanilegbe	Eleggua Barbakikenyer	Eshu Oshanki
Eleggua Agbanile	Eleggua Bilisi	Eshu Oshuni
Eshu Akongoroyo	Eshu Kokogbe	Eshu Okiri
Eshu Alayi Ibere Yeye	Eshu lacerate	Eshu Okuade
Eshu Ala Bono	Eshu LaMeta	Eshu Okueda
Eshu La Bona Ala Gbona	Eshu La Mika	Eshu Okomibade
Eshu Alagbon	Eshu Laye Abaranke	Eshu Onyangui
Eshu Ala Muwa Mubata	Eshu Malu	Eshu Onyankiledo
Eshu Awaya, Aguaya	Eshu Mbemberekete	Eshu Yeku Yelede

In the Congo-derived Afro-Cuban religion Palo Eshu is called Lucero and Kudjo. In Haitian Vodou Eshu's main manifestation is as Papa Legba, but Baron (Bawon) Samedi and the Gede spirits are also aspects of the trickster. To enumerate the many paths of Eshu (Exu) in Brazilian Candomble would require a book dedicated to that alone, but an interesting Brazilian addition to the Eshu catalogue is Pomba Gira, said to be a historical incarnation of Eshu that appeared in Rio at the end of the 19th century as a beautiful prostitute who was stabbed to death. Before she died, a gay man was the only person to come to her aid, so she promised to always look after homosexuals from the land of the spirits. A myth has been told about the great African-American blues singer-guitarist Robert Johnson (d. circa 1937), said to be the best of his genre, about how he sold his soul to the "devil of the crossroads" in order to become the best blues man ever. This story obviously alludes to an African-American cultural retention of an aspect of Eshu that has been transformed into a "devil."

4

ATTRIBUTES

Necklace: Eleggua's traditional necklace, worn by his devotees, consists of alternating red and black beads.[11] Some paths are represented by alternating white and black beads. Black, red, and white beads are also worn for Eleggua. Some traditions play with Eshu's numbers when making his beads, for example, alternating three black/three red beads, or twenty-one black followed by twenty one red beads and so on.

Emblematic colors, numbers, elements, dominions, and Catholic disguised feast days: Eshu's colors are red and black. His principal numbers are one, three, twenty-one, and one hundred-one. A stick off the guava tree in the shape of a cane is one of Eshu-Eleggua's most pervasive attributes. Natalia Bolivar Arostegui says that "Eleggua/Eshu" represent the oriental principle of yin/yang, "the mythic expression of the inevitable connection between positive and negative.[12] Eleggua is the trickster extraordinaire, a Yoruba proverb says "Eshu punishes you today for that which you'll do tomorrow." He has no reverence for linear time and is constantly reminding us how little it means to him.

As The Chief of the Ajogun, agents of misfortune, Eshu reminds us to keep a cool character (iwa pele), the most sought-after quality among the Yoruba, by sending us challenges when we forget to do the right thing. Eshu is the Lord of the Crossroads, which means it is his job to offer us choices. Each time we come to a forked road in our path, it is Eshu who is giving us that choice. By propitiating him before we choose which way to continue, we may be assured a better future. It is said that Eshu creates obstacles in our lives simply to direct our attention to him, like the child he is. Once we make our offering to him, he turns our tragedies into great fortune. Sometimes it is said that Eshu is neither good nor evil, but a neutral force responding to the nature of the sacrifice offered him. He loves abundant offerings, but is also touched by small offerings given with a big heart. Eshu is associated with sexuality and is represented in anthropomorphic fashion as an ithyphallic deity (with an erect penis). Eshu introduced sounding the trumpet to announce great leaders into medieval courts, he also introduced the eating of tortoises into human use. When translated, some of his praise names reveal what Eshu has dominion over, such as "Revealer of Secrets," "Enslaver of People," "Eshu the

Liberator of Slaves," "He-Who-Gives-Fortunes," "He-Who-Takes-Away-Fortunes," "Lord of Communications," "He-Who-Makes-People-Take-Their-Own-Lives," "Lord of Destiny," "Eshu the Carpenter," "Eshu the Gunsmith," "Lord of the Bad Winds," and "He-Who-Makes-Gods-Understandable-To-Humans."

Eshu taught man how to tame the horse, how to build furniture out of wood, how to spin cotton into cloth, how to get fruits out of trees for consumption, and how to use firearms. It is said that Eshu's evil serves to glorify the goodness of God. If God Almighty Olodumare may be said to be the personification of Ashe (primal energy), then Eshu is its guardian, the one who helps Olodumare distribute this primal force to the Orisha, who in turn make the universe move. Without Eshu, there wouldn't be a distribution of Ashe; without Ashe there wouldn't be a dynamic Universe, but one that would experience death through entropy. Eshu's role as the sustainer of order and balance is vital to existence. As Lord of Paradoxes he constantly challenges our minds and our ideas concerning reality. John Wescott perfectly describes Eshu's character in the following note:

> *His Age is reflected in his cunning and in the wisdom concealed in his trickery; his extreme youth in his wantonness and caprice and in his impulsive behavior. Whether old man or child, there is a disregard for the normal code; he enjoys the natural license of the innocent and the privileged license of the aged. As a child, he is the experimenter who breaks rules; as an old man, he enjoys the wisdom that takes him beyond the rules.* [13]

In Cuba Eleggua is syncretized with the Catholic representation of the Baby Jesus known as the Child of Prague, also with the Child of Atocha (Eshu Beleke). He is also syncretized with St. Anthony of Padua (Eshu Laroye) and the Baby Jesus carried by him. Eshu Alabwana is syncretized with the Lonely Soul of Purgatory. Because Eleggua is given the most attention in Santeria, most believers propitiating him every Monday, his feast day is not as widely celebrated as that of other Orisha or, to look at it another way, his feast day is celebrated every Monday! Most Cuban traditions, however, say that his feast days are January 1st, January 6th, and June 13th.

Plants sacred to Eshu Eleggua:

Broadleaf Basil	Fern	Baby's Breath
Guava	Annatto	Tobacco
Camphor	Ebony	Asafetida

Initiation names : At a recent initiation ceremony, during the part of the ritual where a name is given to the initiate, the presiding oriate (master of ceremonies) only remembered a few names. After each name is uttered, the Orisha being enthroned is asked through an oracle if that is to be the name given to the initiate. At this particular ceremony, the oriate ran out of names before the orisha gave a positive answer. Luckily, some of the elders that were present remembered other suitable names and the iyawo did not go home nameless. Respected elder Andres Hing, now residing in Tampa, Florida, published in 1971 the following list of names traditionally given in Cuban Santeria to initiates into the mysteries of Eshu. [14]

Eshu Bi	Eshu Miwa	Osika
Eshu Agulu	Eshu Leti	Aylabode
Eshu Atelu	Eshu Lari	Onibode
Eshu Kilalu	Eshu Akadrede	Bake
Eshu Rine	Eshu Yemi	
Eshu Tolu	Agosede	

Keep this list on hand in order to avoid an embarrassing situation such as the one I described above.

Eshu (Exu) in Brazil: Until relatively recently, the popular media in the United States has tended to ignore Brazil when it carries stories about the Orisha, yet that country has more Orisha-conscious people than any other nation in the world! It is perhaps due to the tenacity with which practitioners of Candomble, their equivalent of Santeria, guard their traditions there, and their reluctance to initiate people outside of Brazil, that they have been able to maintain such a low profile. This state of affairs, however, is quickly changing as all aspects of Orisha worship are coming under media scrutiny, due to increased public interest in Orisha culture in general, and also due to more Brazilian-made priests becoming more visible in the U.S. Artist Manny Vega, for example, whose mosaics depicting Yemaya and Shango adorns the 110th street subway station on the 6 line in New York City, throws a fabulous, star-studded party every year to celebrate his anniversary as a priest of Oxossi.

Brazilian scholar Nunes Pereira calls Exu a "gigantic, dynamic, and disorienting personality."[15] Arne Falke Ronne describes Exu as an "insaciable erotic, able to satisfy 3,500 women in a 24 hour period.[16] The premier recorder of Afro-Brazilian life, Franco-Brazilian anthropologist Roger Bastide, who "went native" (became an initiate), says of Exu: "His function is to regulate the cosmos. It is he who blocks all pathways and removes all obstacles. In effect, he is the God of Order."[17]

Some of the Brazilian Exus (besides Pomba Gira, discussed above) include Arranca-Toco, Tranca Ruas, Male, Tiriri, Caveira, Brasa, Marabo, Veludo, Pemba, Mirim, Carangola, Maria Padilha, Quebra-Galho, Mangeira, Giramundo, Ze Pelintra, and Pedra Negra. In Brazil Exu is often depicted as a Mephistophelian devil, complete with horns, pointed beard, and long, black cape. He is also syncretized with St. Anthony and St. Peter in Porto Alegre, and with St. Gabriel the Archangel in Recife.

Shrine (Igbodu): *How initiates honor Eshu Eleggua:* As one of the "Warriors," a group of four Orisha most serious followers of Santeria receive, even if they do not go all the way into full initiation into the mysteries of their tutelary deity in the kariosha ceremony. Some, however, are children of Eshu and receive his mysteries directly on their heads. Eshu's initiations, then, fall basically into two categories: The mid-level initiation called *"The Warriors,"* and the high-level initiation known as *"Kariosha,"* or *"Making the Saint."* This means that Eshu, like other Orisha, has his own egbe (denomination); yet he is also worshipped across the board in all egbes, since members of all other cults have to have received the preliminary initiation of the Warriors before they can go on to receive full initiation.

The Warriors consist of an Eleggua image, generally depicted in one of the following three forms: As a small cement cone with eyes, nose, mouth, and ears fashioned out of cowry shells; this figure rests in a small terra cotta or earthenware dish; as a conch filled with cement with features made out of cowry shells; and as a natural stone that has been consecrated. Wood Elegguas are also sometimes employed. The next orisha to be conferred as part of the warriors is Ogun, Lord of War and of Iron. He is represented by a black, three-legged iron pot filled with railroad spikes, horseshoes, a stone consecrated to Ogun, and iron implements such as a miniature plow, a sword, a hoe, etc. Inside Ogun's pot, Oshosi, Lord of the Hunt and the Divine Tracker, is represented with his own stone and with an iron bow-and-arrow. The fourth Orisha in the Warriors group is Osun, pronounced oh-SOON, represented by a metal chalice fringed with jingle bells and topped by a rooster. Many writers have equated Osun with Osanyin, but those of us steeped in Cuban Santeria know these are completely different Orisha. Osun seems to be of Arara origin. He represents the initiate as his physical presence in the Warriors group. When the Osun chalice falls down, the initiate breaks an egg over it and becomes aware that something serious, possibly troublesome, is to happen unless proper steps are taken. Those who have not undergone the kariosha initiation can communicate with Eleggua and the other warriors through the use of the Obi oracle. According to Yoruba tradition, this is an utterly egalitarian oracle; no initiation is necessary in order to access its wisdom. (see next chapter). The Warriors should be kept close to the home's main entrance (front door). Some people place them inside a foot locker or some other large container in order to guard their own, as well as the Warriors', privacy. Those who have Eleggua as their tutelary (head) deity and have undergone Kariosha have much more elaborate shrines dedicated to their Orisha. These shrines may feature fine curtains of red and black material, fancy porcelain soup tureens holding Eleggua's 21 cowry shells, and embroidered clothes depicting Catholic icons related to the worship of Eleggua.

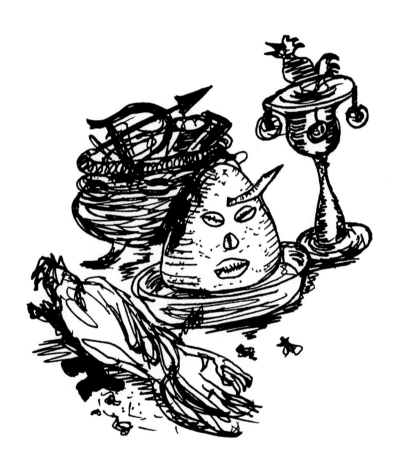

Warriors with rooster offering

Shrine (ojubo alejo) How non-initiates may honor Eshu Eleggua: Many homes in Cuba feature a small altar to the Child of Prague, or a statue of St. Anthony, or a print of the Lonely Souls, a medieval representation of a beautiful woman burning in a fiery inferno, close to the front door. A coconut placed on a white plate behind the front door of many homes is also used to represent Eleggua in households that don't have initiates.

Minor offerings (adimu): Eshu likes everything children like: toys, candies, coloring pencils etc. He also likes to be adorned with the red tail feathers of the African gray parrot. The more grave aspects of Eshu like hot peppers. All Eshus like to be dressed with palm oil, which is deep orange or red. They also like coffee, rum, toasted corn, smoked jutia (a large rodent that looks like an opossum), smoked fish, sugar cane, eggs, kola nuts, cascarilla chalk, coconut juice, fresh water, pieces of fabric, and cigar smoke. All Eshus hate corn kernel oil, which is yellow. In fact, a very dangerous spell, one I wouldn't recommend, is to offer Eshu red palm oil saying "I, so-and-so, give you this palm oil," then, you would spread palm kernel oil over his cowry shell mouth while saying the name of an enemy you want to destroy in the following fashion: "so-and-so gives you this corn kernel oil." Eshu gets so upset that he kills whoever you mentioned. Eshu also hates squash and does not allow menstruating women to work with him while on their menses.

Major offerings (ebo): Jutia (a large Cuban rodent) is Eshu's favorite offering. In North America he accepts rats, mice, guinea pigs, and opossums as substitutes. Eshu also likes roosters, chickens, and newly-hatched chicks, deer, goats, dogs, and tortoises. Some Eshus accept pigeon sacrifices (must be two at a time), but most do not.

Characteristics of Eshu's devotees (sons and daughters): Eshu's children tend to be intelligent and cunning. They are prone to perpetrate practical jokes on whoever makes a suitable victim. They are also sexually diverse and outside what the majority of people would call "normal." Politicians, clowns, and tollkeepers are protected by Eleggua, as are thieves and other underworld characters.

5

OBI:
HOW TO COMMUNICATE WITH THE
GREAT COMMUNICATOR

How Eshu Eleggua made it possible for everyone to have access to the Obi oracle: The following pataki tells the story of Obi, the Orisha who, because of false pride, was downgraded to common oracle. Eshu-Eleggua was responsible for Obi's downfall by reporting Obi's misbehavior to their father, Olofi. In this manner, an Orisha's disgrace became humanity's gain, a pattern Eshu-Eleggua would repeat with Ogun, whose own downfall made it possible for humankind to obtain the secret of forging iron.

During the time when the orisha and humankind still lived together, Olofi's son Obi was made to rule over a vast domain that included both orisha and men. A beautiful youth fond of wearing impeccable white garments like his father, Obi was a kind and careful ruler. So popular did Obi become that potentates from all over would come to praise the young prince. At first he took equal delight in welcoming humble fishermen and even lepers, as well as princes and rich merchants, into his presence. But slowly, Prince Obi's head began to swell, and he became proud and snobbish. At a public party, where all his subjects were supposed to be welcome, Obi gave orders not to let "the lower classes" in. Disguised as a beggar, Obi's brother Eshu-Eleggua attempted to enter the party, only to be physically ejected by Prince Obi's guards.

Eshu ran to Olofi, telling the Great God what Prince Obi was doing. Olofi also disguised himself as a poor man and, joining Eshu, attempted to enter the party. This time Prince Obi himself happened to be near the gate when he saw the two paupers attempting to enter. "Please, noble Prince, give us some crumbs off your table," a disguised Eshu pleaded. "Be gone with you, riffraff, how dare you think I would talk to such filth!" At that moment both Eshu's and Olofin's rags fell down, revealing the Old emperor's exquisite silver robes and Eshu's delightful silk gowns. Realizing who the two were, Obi fell to the ground crying, begging Olofin to forgive him. Raising his right arm, Olofin cursed Obi thus: "From now on that magnificent brightness you are so proud of exhibiting will be inside you, your outside being dark and hairy, dirty and coarse. You will continually fall from palms and children will kick you for sport. Your great wisdom will be accessible to anyone who asks, so you will serve everyone as an oracle."

This is the reason people use coconuts as oracles, but must always act respectfully towards these fruits, asking permission before breaking them down to make the Obi oracle. Although Obi was punished, he was a great prince and an orisha, so we must look upon the coconut with great respect.

The place of oracles in Santeria's belief system: An extremely important function of Eshu is as the God of Oracles, especially the Obi oracle, which in Cuba is synonymous with coconut, itself a manifestation of Eshu-Eleggua in many traditions, and an oracle that does not require initiation to be performed. Before expounding on the Obi oracle, let us examine the cross-cultural phenomenon of divination itself: What is divination?: It is the manipulation of religious symbols as a problem-solving process. Most divination systems use certain transcendent or metaphysical images which are then manipulated to give illumination on a problem or a particular situation. In Africa, there are two main systems of divination. One involves the manipulation of shells, nuts, or rocks. The other is to mark symbols on the earth and then either let animals loose to walk upon them, or wait for wild animals to spontaneously walk across them. There are, of course, other systems of divination in Africa, such as water-gazing and spirit possession, but the first two I have described are the most widely employed.

As an issue of faith, or belief, when divination is used it is our belief that divination is effective because the selection process is inspired and/or guided by benevolent, superior, Spiritual Forces. In this manner, divination is not only the manipulation of metaphysical symbols, but also a way of achieving direct communication with Forces of Nature. This you either believe, or you do not. "Proving" it one way or the other is hard, to put it mildly. Coming back to Jung, he performed studies on divination systems and came up with the concept of synchronization to explain why divination works. Synchronization refers to two seemingly unrelated events having an underlying meaning. Behind the concept of synchronization is the belief that the entire universe is interrelated. This is a typically African concept, the belief that nothing can happen unconnected to anything else. Another explanation of why divination works is that it is a form of mind-over-matter. Or the closely related concept of wish-fulfillment. You are told by a Gypsy that you'll die on your 60th birthday, so when that date arrives, you may inadvertently cause your own death, thereby fulfilling the prophecy. In Santeria we believe divination is a form of direct communication with Spiritual Forces. Traditionally, the Yoruba have counted on four main systems of communication with their Higher Spirits. One is divination, one is possession, one is dreams, and the fourth is interpretation of signs in nature. Divination can be very complex, as exemplified by the complicated system known as the oracle of Ifa, which involves the casting of a chain or manipulation of palm nuts in order to obtain a sign, called an odu which is notated as eight marks, each representing light (I), or darkness (II). An odu looks like this:

$$
\begin{array}{cc}
\mathbf{I} & \mathbf{I} \\
\mathbf{II} & \mathbf{II} \\
\mathbf{II} & \mathbf{I} \\
\mathbf{II} & \mathbf{II}
\end{array}
$$

In the Ifa system, each "throw" of the divining chain gives you eight positions with two possible marks for each, thus manifesting one of 256 possible configurations, each called an "odu." Notice the similarity of this system with the Chinese I Ching system. Ifa, however, is much more intricate. According to the distinguished American babalawo and theologian, Awo Falokun, the word "odu" means womb. In his lucid exposition on Ifa, Falokun states that each odu is to be regarded as a fundamental energy pattern that sustains creation on all the different dimensions of being. Each odu is said to contain twelve different possible interpretations, thus giving the diviner 3,072 possible answers to each single question. Obviously, mastering such a mind-boggling amount of information requires a lifetime of dedication. Also, remember that traditionally babalawo were expected to master this system mentally, without the aid of written materials. In fact, although the Ifa system of divination may be thousands of years old, attempts to write down its wisdom can be traced back no more than two-hundred years.

In Africa, a boy would be chosen by divination at the age of seven to begin to study under an elder. For the next seven years, the apprentice was expected to memorize all 256 odu. After demonstrating that they had attained this goal, the 14 year old apprentices could then be initiated into the mysteries of Ifa. They were then expected to spend the rest of their lives mastering the oracle. Because of the dedication required to become a proficient babalawo, Ifa diviners enjoy great prestige in Yoruba society. In Cuban Santeria, though the requirements for babalawo are not nearly as demanding, they are afforded great respect and act as de-facto high priests in the religion. Only babalawo are thought to have the necessary Ashe (grace) to cast the oracle, so non-initiates should not attempt to do so.

Next in complexity among Yoruba oracles is merindilogun, also known as the Sixteen Cowry divination system. The relationship of the cowry shall oracle to Ifa is complicated, for although even Wande Abimbola, the international spokesman for Ifa among all nations, admits that merindilogun is older than Ifa, babalawo tend to look down on this system as not being nearly as systematized and catalogued as Ifa. Any initiate into the priesthood of any orisha can learn how to throw the shells, unless prohibited by their own initiatory reading (ita) to do so.

Thanks to Eshu-Eleggua, the simplest oracle, the Obi oracle, is open to everyone! Greedy practitioners of Santeria have maintained that only priests and priestesses can perform Obi divination. Most santeros do not teach their godchildren the art of coconut casting. This is a reprehensible situation, since Obi is a way of connecting with the ancestors and with Eshu. Since everyone has ancestors, everyone has a right to learn Obi divination.

To ensure the success of divination, we should perform it in a sacred space, an area that is designated, consecrated, and only used for the purpose of divination. The traditional way for this to be done is by designating a straw mat as the sacred space, thus we can carry our sacred space with us wherever we go!

Next, we should bring the elements of earth, air, fire, and water to the divining mat. All we need to add is a candle and a glass of water, for earth and air are already present. In Africa, Obi divination is done with four pieces of kola nut. In America, we use four pieces of coconut. Both kola nuts and coconuts are considered intrinsically holy and imbued with mystical powers. Some people use four cowry shells I often use permakolas®, an object of divination I developed based on West African coastal traditions, where pieces of consecrated kola nuts are mixed with clay, formed into two-inch squares or circles, and baked until hard. Sometimes a cowry shell is embedded on one side to differentiate the "heads" from the "tails." The complex prayer that is recited at the beginning of each divination session has been simplified here to help the beginner.

Mo juba Olodumare, Olorun, Olofi.
Mo juba Egun mi.
Mo juba (insert name of dead ancestor)
Mo juba (name another ancestor, etc.)
Maferefun Eshu
Maferefun Ogun
Maferefun Oshosi
Maferefun Osun
Maferefun Obatala
Maferefun Shango, Kabio Sile!
Maferefun Orunla
Maferefun Aganju
Maferefun Yemaya
Maferefun Oya

Maferefun Oshun
Maferefun Yewa
Maferefun Dada
Maferefun Nana Bukuu
Maferefun Orishaoko
Maferefun gbogbo orisha!

Ona tutu
Ile tutu
Ori tutu
Laroye tutu

(repeat 3 times from "Ona tutu...", pouring a bit of water on the ground each time)

KinkamashéBaba Raul Canizares
(or any elder you feel connected with)
Kinkamashé all elders, brothers, and sisters in Osha.
Kinkamashé to my godchildren (if applicable)

Ko si Iku
Ko si Arun
Ko si Epe
Ko si Oran
Ko si Ofo
Ko Si Araye
Ko Si Ashelu
Ko Si Fitibo
Ko Si Egba
Ko Si Ewan
Ko si Eshe

Fun mi ni Alafia
Fun mi ni owo
Fun mi ni ire
Fun mi ni tutu
Fun mi ni ilera
Ashé!

Translation:

Praises to God Almighty
Praises to all my ancestors
Praises to so-and-so(name an ancestor)
May Eshu's name be honored
May Ogun's name be honored
May Oshosi's name be honored
etc.,
May all orisha be honored!

May my road be fresh and clear
May my home be fresh and clear
May my head be fresh and clear
May the orisha of communications be fresh and clear

Praises to Baba Raul Canizares
(or any elder you feel connected with)
Praises to all elders, brothers etc.,

Keep away death
Keep away sickness
Keep away curses
Keep away big trouble
Keep away loss
Keep away tragedy
Keep away injustice
Keep away small obstacles

Keep away paralysis
Keep away prison
Keep away all else that is bad for me

May I receive peace
May I receive money
May I receive grace
May I receive clarity and freshness
May I receive a stable home life
So be it!

We are now ready to divine! The four pieces that make up the Obi oracle give five major answers depending on how many land face up or face down. Whether it is the white, pulpy side of a coconut piece or the side marked by a cowry shell in a permakola, we'll call this side the "white" side, calling the other side the "dark" side. The five main answers of Obi are:

0 0 0 0 - Alafia

When all four pieces fall white side up, the answer is "Alafia." This is a "yes" with blessings. It could also mean an unexpected yes. When Alafia comes up, all present must touch the ground with the points of three fingers of the right hand, immediately kissing them. Generally a good omen, it can be tricky sometimes. This is why learned readers do not consider "Alafia" to be a definite "yes." Case in point is that of a godchild of mine who asked if when the returned from a trip his ailing mother would be doing better. The answer he got was Alafia, which he interpreted as being yes. When he returned from his trip, my godson found his mother dead. By not suffering, she was indeed doing "better," but this was certainly not what he had expected. I recommend that when Alafia comes out, do not take it as a simple yes, rather, view it in a more all-encompassing light and perhaps follow it with a couple of clarifying questions.

0 0 0 ● - Itawa

Three whites up. Generally considered a weak "yes,"[18] it demands a follow-up throw. If second throw is *Alafia,* answer is "yes, with blessings!" If follow-up throw is *Itawa* again, the answer is "yes, after some initial difficulties." If follow-up is *Ejife,* answer is "yes, but calm down a bit." If *Okana* comes up on second throw, answer is "abandon question, a yes could be dangerous" or "a hollow victory not worth your time and energy."

0 0 ● ● - Ejife

Two up, two down; a definite **YES.**

0 ● ● ● - Okana

One white up, three down. A definite **NO.**

● ● ● ● - Oyeku

All whites down. An indication that a more sophisticated oracle needs to be consulted, for the matter at hand is way too complicated to be reduced to a "yes" or "no" format. When Oyeku comes up, all four pieces of the oracle need to be immersed in water. If Oyeku comes up three or more times during a reading, the person being read is definitely in need of a more thorough consultation with an elder, since Oyeku persistently popping up is a strong indication of very complex questions needing equally complex solutions beyond the scope of the Obi oracle.

The key to obtaining accurate information from the Obi oracle rests in your ability to frame questions properly. Following some simple rules will ensure success. Non-initiates may address their questions to "my spirit guides," specific spirits known to them as guides (always ask `will you answer my questions?' in this case), or to Eshu-Eleggua.

1: Always frame your question in a manner that can be answered "yes" or "no"--example: *"Am I getting the job of supervisor this week when it becomes available?"* It is important that you put a time frame on your question whenever possible, because if you merely ask Will I get the job of supervisor?" The oracle may give a "yes" based on the fact that you will become a supervisor ten years down the line!

2: Avoid ambiguities: frame your question *"Does J.D. feel erotic love for me?"* rather than "Does J.D. love me?" J.D. may love you like a son, but that's NOT what you are hoping for.

3: Avoid double negatives such as "Does Mark not feel what he doesn't feel for me?"

4: Although there is a rule that once you have obtained an answer you do not ask the same question again, you may cross-reference an answer to make sure of its accuracy. This must be done one after the other for less confusion. Example-- *"Does Jeannie feel erotic love for me?"* Immediately followed by "Is Jeannie aware that she is sexually attracted to me?"

5: Think of relevant and pertinent follow-up questions such as *"Will getting together with Jeannie in a romantic relationship be advantageous and relatively worthwhile for me?"* and *"Will getting together with me be relatively good for Jeannie?"*

6: There is a very important Yoruba proverb that says "If you already know the answer, don't ask the question." This literally means that the oracle does not respond well to frivolous questions. For example, if you truly KNOW your husband finds you attractive, don't ask *"Does my husband find me attractive?"* Because the oracle will give you a nonsense response.

7: Be as specific as possible: example-- *"Will I pass the math test on Thursday?"* Rather than "Will I do well in math?"

Following these guidelines will ensure your
divination will be remarkably accurate.

Once the five principal answers are mastered, other, more subtle additional meanings can be gleamed from the way the pieces fall. For example, if a white falls directly on top of another white, this indicates a surge of good fortune associated with the question.

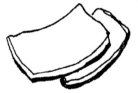

If a white falls on top of a dark, this indicates an end to bad luck coming about due to some variable associated with the question.

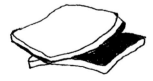

A dark falling on top of a dark indicates an advent of bad fortune.

A dark falling on top of a white indicates that steps must be taken to ensure the success of whatever is being considered.

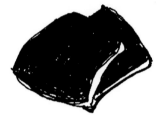 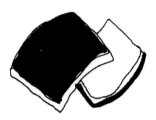

If a single piece falls out of your hand while you are about to execute a throw, this means the spirit answering is in a rush to communicate. If the piece falls white side up, the answer is "yes".

If the piece falls white side down, the answer is "no".

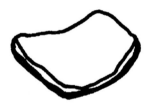 

If one of the pieces falls standing on its edge, a spirit guide is present and wants to communicate at a level higher than the obi oracle.

6

Eshu - Eleggua
and Santeria's
"CELESTIAL COURT"

In Africa, orisha worshippers generally belong to a society ("egbe") dedicated to the worship of a single orisha, thus, worshippers of Aganju would belong to egbe Aganju, those who worship Yemaya would belong to egbe Yemaya and so forth. These societies were in fact denominations, fully self-sufficient and not necessarily having anything to do with initiations into orishas other than their own. The three elements of orisha worship that transcended the boundaries of egbe were Eshu worship, ancestor veneration ("egungun") and Ifa divination. Eshu-Eleggua is worshipped across the board because of reasons we have already discussed, mainly, that as the orisha who opens and closes doors, both literal and metaphysical, he can keep anyone from achieving anything. The ancestors, of course, form the backbone of most indigenous spiritualities, for it is in great part deified ancestors who receive the greatest amount of worship in many of these primal[19] societies. Ifa priests have attained great fame and respect as codifiers, recorders, and teachers of orisha worship. Although strictly speaking they are one more egbe among many, in reality they are the scholars of orisha worship and have attained the status of high priests. In Santeria there is a saying which goes: "Everyone ends up at the feet of Orunla," meaning that sooner or later, most practitioners in Africa and Cuba--not so in Brazil, where there are not many babalawo--have to resort to Ifa divination to settle disputes. The wife of a babalawo (Ifa practitioner) is usually a priestess herself, ideally of Oshun. Although she shouldn't cast cowries or engage in divination, she can perform all priestly duties including initiating others and having her own godchildren.

During the shameful days of the slave trade, members of all egbes were criminally brought to the Americas. Under the horrible conditions endured by these incredibly brave men, women, and children, they found their lives interrupted in a fashion so lacking in humanity that it is hard for us today to imagine how our ancestors were able to withstand being subjected to such ignominy just a few generations ago. Members of different egbe would be grouped together in different plantations. Lacking the infrastructures they had enjoyed in their homeland, egbes that in Africa would have nothing to do with each other became associated by necessity. A member of egbe Oshun, for example, would teach a member of egbe Shango about his religion, while the member of Shango's egbe would reciprocate. In this fashion, each worshipper made sure his or her orisha would not fall into oblivion. Eventually, a synthesis began to occur where the egbes began to become fused into a single religion, Lukumi, also called "Regla de Ocha" and Santeria.

Where the ashe of a single orisha would be revealed to an initiate in Africa, a standard five orisha were offered automatically in a Santeria initiation, though only one of these would be installed in a person's head. The five standard orishas were: Eshu (Eleggua), Obatala, Shango, Yemaya, and Oshun.

Cuban elders refer to the Santeria pantheon as "La Corte Celestial," the Celestial Court. Eshu-Eleggua's position in the pantheon is unique. He is the only orisha all egbes had to honor in Africa, a custom that survived the Middle Passage. In Santeria, receiving the mid-level Warriors initiation is mandatory for all serious devotees. As head warrior, Eshu is in all the homes of orisha worshippers around the globe. Eshu-Eleggua is also carried by devotees, small "pocket Elegguas" being fashioned out of small shells and other materials many times. Also, each orisha conferred generally has his or her own Eshu. Thus, when one receives Babalu, one also needs Eshu Afra.

Although orisha worship continued to develop separately in Yorubaland in Africa and in Cuba, one aspect of the religion that has continued to be expressed with remarkable consistency is Eshu Eleggua's primacy over all other Orisha, his virtual ubiquity in all ceremonies concerning the Orisha, and his unique relationship to God, the Orisha, and Humankind, as the force that keeps the Universe moving.

7

ORIKI ESHU ELEGGUA;
ORIN ESHU ELEGGUA
PRAYERS AND SONGS TO ESHU ELEGGUA

PRAISE POEMS TO ESHU-ELEGGUA (ORIKI)

Eshu turns right into wrong, wrong into right.
When he is angry, he hits a stone until it bleeds.
When he is angry, he sits on the skin of an ant.
When he is angry, he weeps tears of blood.

Eshu slept in the house-
but the house was too small for him.
Eshu slept on the verandah-
but the verandah was too small for him.
Eshu slept in a nut-
at last he could stretch himself.

Eshu walked through the groundnut farm.
The tuft of his hair was just visible.
If it had not been for his huge size,
he would not be visible at all.
Lying down, his head hits the roof.
Standing up, he cannot look into the cooking pot.
He throws a stone today and kills a bird yesterday?[20]

II

Owner and elder of the crossroads. My father, remove all evil, for us to
walk in peace, loss is no more, tragedy is no more, sickness is no more,
death is no more, unforseen evil is no more, in the name of all children
in this house, I give you thanks, my father Elegba.[21]

III

Your friends are those who offer you respect.
Your enemies are those who do not know your worth, and do not feed you

You own no farm or market, Your farm is the entire universe.
Your merchandise, Olodumare's creation. [22]

IV

Here is Exu, midnight Exu Exu of intersections! Here are Exu and his wife, the
lovely Pomba-Gira! He's wearing his black cape he's wearing his black hat he's
wearing his polished shoes. With his iron trident in his hand, Here is Exu
midnight Exu, Exu of intersections! [23]

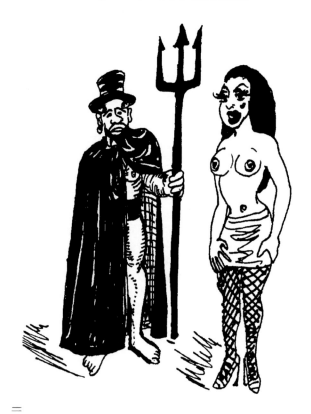

=

V

Na escuridão da noite magica,
Exu crava na encruzilhada sete espadas,
que são os sete caminhos do seu império.
Logo vem encontra-lo seu irmão Ogum.
E partem ambos pelas sendas do desconhecido,
a servico dos deuces a dos mortais![24]

In the darkness of a magical night,
Eshu plants seven swords at the crossroads,
that represent the seven paths of his empire.
He goes on to meet his brother Ogun,
and both continue on their journey through unknown trails,
at the service of gods and mortals alike! [25]

Praise Songs to Eshu-Eleggua (orin)

I

Barasuwayo, Omoni Alawana, mamakenya irawo Eee
*(Eshu of mischief who gives Oyo its Character, Child who owns the crossroads,
do not cut mother, the stars praise you)*

O Barasuwayo, Eee
(Eshu of mischief; who gives Oyo its Character, be praised)

Eshu Odara, Omoni Alawana, Mamakenya irawo, Fee
*(Eshu the Criminal, Child who owns the crossroads, do not cut mother,
the stars praise you)*

Lord of Mischief, you give character to Oyo. Child who owns the crossroads, do
not let any harm come to our mothers, the stars in heaven sing your praises.

Great Lord of Mischief, we praise you, Eshu the Criminal, Child who owns the
crossroads, do not let any harm come to our mothers, the stars in heaven sing
your praise!

II

Ibara ago mo juba
(Mischief, give way, I praise you)

Ibara ago, ago mo juba
(Mischief, give way, I praise you greatly)

Omode Koniko
(Crowned Child who teaches doctrine)

Ibara ago mojuba
(Mischief, give way, I praise you)

Elegba 'ku L'ona
(Elegba, move death away from my path)

III

Ago Elegba o bu kenke
(Make way for Elegba who is abusive and small)

Ago laroye o bu kenke
(Make way for Laroye who is abusive and small)

Ago Elegba o bu kenke
(Make way for Elegba who is abusive and small)

Ago laroye o bu kenke
(Make way for Laroye who is abusive and small) [26]

---

[1] Carl Gustav Jung (1875-1961) was a pioneering and visionary psychoanalyst whose influence extended far beyond his field.

[2] Although many respected scholars, including Awo 'Falokun and John Mason, translate the word "orisha" as "select head," Wande Abimbola, foremost spokesman for Yoruba religion in the world, emphatically states that this is a mistake. He translates the word as "Something that you plant on the ground and to which you have to pay homage." See Ifa *Will Mend Our Broken* World, Pp. 154-155.

[3] Although it is commonly believed that Eshu is the first orisha to partake of the blood of sacrificed animals, in reality Ogun receives any sacrifice first. This is due to the fact that Ogun is the life-force of any being, and when that life-force is released, Ogun automatically partakes of it.

[4] As an example see the glossary in back of Julio Garcia-Cortez's influential manual El *Santo, La Ocha* (Mexico: Editora Latino Americana, 1976), page 561, where the spelling for "ewe" is given as "egue."

[5] Like the word "Orisha," the word "pataki" does not change in the plural. Some writers do use "patakis" or "patakies" when speaking of pataki in the plural.

[6] A version of this pataki is found in Garcia-Cortez, p. 107.

[7] Although many practitioners, particularly in the U.S., believe Osun and Osanyin are equivalent, this is totally mistaken. They are totally different orisha.

[8] Although the story of Ogun's incest is not told in modern-day Nigeria, but it has been told in Cuba since at least the 1800's, I suspect the story has been suppressed in Africa due to Ogun's growing role as a paragon of justice and truth.

[9] In Cuba Oya is thought to live in the cemetery gates, where she receives the corpses that Babalu Aiye brings there. In Africa, Oya's position as patron orisha of the egungun society also has her in close contact with death.

[10] The Arara formed the fourth major Afro-Cuban ethno-religious group, the other three being the Lukumi (Yoruba), Palo Mayombe (Congo), and Abakua (Efik). Arara seems to be a mispronunciation of Alladha, a city in modern Benin.

[11] In large American cities such as Los Angeles and New York, many santeros are no longer using this pattern because identical red and black beaded necklaces are used by certain gangs as a sign of membership. The red, black, and white being preferred.

[12] My translation of "la expresion mitica de la inevitable relation entre to positivo y to negativo" p. 36.

[13] See Joan Wescott, "The Sculpture and Myths of Eshu-Elegba, The Yoruba trickster-Definition and Interpretation In Yoruba Iconography". Africa, Vol. 32 (1962), pp. 336353.

[14] Andres Hing. Oddun de Ifa al Caracol " Self-Published, 1971.

[15] Quoted in Sangirardi Jr., Deuses da Africa a do Brazil: Candomble a Umbanda (Brasilia: Editora Civilizacao Brasileira, 1988) p. 77.

[16] ibid.

[17] ibid.

[18] In most Ifa houses, itawa is a definite "yes."

[19] I am using "primal" here not to imply "primitive," but "primary," "first."

[20] Ully Beier, Yoruba Poetry (Cambridge: Cambridge University Press, 1970), p.28.

[21] Anthony Ferreira, Eshu Osanyin (Brooklyn, N.Y.: Athelia Henrietta Press, 2000), p. 1-B.

[22] Souza, Op.Cit., p.17.

[23] Serge Bramly, Macumba (Monroe, Oregon: City Lights Press, 1994) p. 192.

[24] Sangirardi Jr,. Op Cit, p. 67

[25] My translation.

[26] John Mason, Orin Orisa (Brooklyn: Y.T.A., 1992) p. 72.

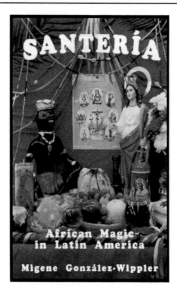

ITEM #001
$14.95

SANTERIA
AFRICAN MAGIC
IN LATIN AMERICA

BY MIGENE GONZALEZ WIPPLER

In 1973, the first hardcover edition of *Santeria: African Magic in Latin America* by cultural anthropologist Migene Gonzalez-Wippler was first published by Julian Press. It became an immediate best-seller and is still considered by many experts one of the most popular books on Santeria, having gone through 4 editions and several translations. Now this beloved classic, written by one the foremost scholars on the Afro-Cuban religion, has returned in a 5th edition. This time the text has been carefully edited and corrected to incorporate vital new material. The beliefs, practices, legends of Santeria are brilliantly brought to life in this exciting and critically acclaimed best-seller. If you ever wondered what Santeria is, if you are curious about the rituals and practices of this mysterious religion, and want to delve in its deepest secrets, this book will answer all your questions and much more.

ISBN 0-942272-04-8 5½"x 8½" $14.95

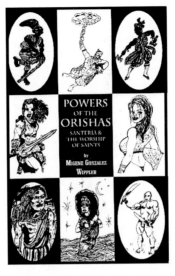

POWERS OF THE ORISHAS
Santeria and the Worship of Saints
Migene Gonzalez Wippler

Santeria is the Afro-Cuban religion based on an amalgamation between some of the magio-religious beliefs and practices of the Yoruba people and those of the Catholic church. In Cuba where the Yoruba proliferated extensively, they became known as *Lucumi,* a word that means "friendship".

Santeria is known in Cuba as Lucumi Religion. The original Yoruba language, interspersed with Spanish terms and corrupted through the centuries of misuse and mispronunciation, also became known as Lucumi. Today some of the terms used in Santeria would not be recognized as Yoruba in Southwestern Nigeria, the country of origin of the Yoruba people.

Santeria is a Spanish term that means a confluence of saints and their worship. These saints are in reality clever disguises for some of the Yoruba deities, known as Orishas. During the slave trade, the Yoruba who were brought to Cuba were forbidden the practice of their religion by their Spanish masters. In order to continue their magical and religious observances safely the slaves opted for the identification and disguise of the Orishas with some of the Catholic saints worshipped by the Spaniards. In this manner they were able to worship their deities under the very noses of the Spaniards without danger of punishment.

Throughout the centuries the practices of the Yoruba became very popular and soon many other people of the Americas began to practice the new religion.

ISBN 0-942272-25-0 5½"x 8½" 144 pages $9.95